Award ... thor
of nu ... d by
the press as the gur ... most
original voice in health'. A shining example of energy and
commitment, she is highly respected for her thorough
reporting. Leslie was born in California, and is the daughter
of jazz musician Stan Kenton. After leaving Stanford
University she journeyed to Europe in her early twenties,
settling first in Paris, then in Britain, where she has since
remained. She has raised four children on her own by
working as a television broadcaster, novelist, writer and
teacher on health and for fourteen years she was an editor
at *Harpers & Queen*.

Leslie's writing on mainstream health is internationally
known and has appeared in *Vogue*, *The Sunday Times*,
Cosmopolitan and the *Daily Mail*. She is author of many
other health books including: *The New Raw Energy*, *Raw
Energy Recipes* and *Endless Energy* – co-authored with her
daughter Susannah – *The New Biogenic Diet*, *The New Joy of
Beauty*, *The New Ageless Ageing*, *Cellulite Revolution*, *10 Day
Clean-Up Plan*, *Nature's Child*, *Lean Revolution*, *10 Day
De-Stress Plan*, *Passage to Power* and most recently, *Raw
Energy Food Combining Diet* and *Juice High*. She turned to
fiction with *Ludwig* – her first novel. Former consultant to a
medical corporation in the USA and to the Open
University's Centre of Continuing Education, Leslie's
writing has won several awards including the PPA
'Technical Writer of the Year'. Her work was honoured by
her being asked to deliver the McCarrison Lecture at the
Royal Society of Medicine. In recent years she has become
increasingly concerned not only with the process of
enhancing individual health but also with re-establishing
bonds with the earth as part of helping to heal the planet.

Get Fit

LESLIE KENTON

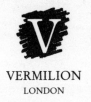

VERMILION
LONDON

1 3 5 7 9 10 8 6 4 2

First published in the United Kingdom in 1996
by Vermilion
an imprint of Ebury Press
Random House
20 Vauxhall Bridge Road
London SW1V 2SA

Random House Australia (Pty) Limited
20 Alfred Street, Milsons Point, Sydney,
New South Wales 2061, Australia

Random House New Zealand Limited
18 Poland Road, Glenfield,
Auckland 10, New Zealand

Random House South Africa (Pty) Limited
PO BOX 337, Bergvlei, South Africa

Random House Canada
1265 Aerowood Drive, Mississauga
Ontario L4W 1B9, Canada

Random House UK Limited Reg. No. 954009

A CIP catalogue record for this book is available from the
British Library

ISBN: 0 09 181450 2

Printed and bound in Great Britain by
Cox & Wyman Ltd., Reading, Berkshire

Contents

chapter 1

What is Fitness?

Introduction

When you are really fit you will be strong, supple and have stamina. *Strength* is muscle power – the extra push that makes you able to deal with unexpected heavy tasks like pushing a car or lifting a heavy load. *Suppleness* is flexibility, the ability to bend and stretch freely without pain and to twist and turn as you wish. Being supple is being mobile, so you can reach up high for things on a shelf, squat down easily, or sit comfortably in a chair or on the floor for long periods. Your body will stay supple if you use all of its muscles and joints regularly. If you don't you will get stiff and feel old. The notion that because you may be approaching forty or fifty or sixty you can *expect* to get stiff is nonsense. Stiffness at any age can be prevented through a diet low in fat and moderate in protein and high in fresh raw foods, combined with proper exercise.

And what is *stamina*? Stamina is endurance, staying power, the ability to work hard and long without fatigue – not only physical stamina, but mental and emotional stamina too. In order to build both strength and stamina you need to put your body's large groups of muscles – those muscles in your legs and arms, for instance – through their paces and challenge your heart and lungs.

Keep it simple

You certainly don't have to be an athlete to achieve a high level of fitness and health. In fact, studies show that the excessive training and stress to which athletes subject their bodies can be counter-productive.

Excessive exercise can undermine the immune system, cause loss of muscle from bones and make you age rapidly. When it comes to using exercise to promote health, the goal is not to become a 'sports nut' but just to create an active lifestyle for yourself and then to stick to it. Neither do you need a lot of special equipment. Exercise has become the latest and greatest commodity in our consumer-fixated culture and the fast-growing exercise industry is becoming highly sophisticated, selling exorbitantly expensive para-phernalia from computerized bicycles to automatic treadmills and you require none of it to get the benefits of fitness. All that is really needed is motivation, some active involvement and a determination to rearrange your lifestyle so you can fit it all in.

Check it out

To help determine just how fit you are at the present moment here is a check list. How many of the questions below you can answer 'yes' to? How many get a 'no'?

- Do you tire after carrying a couple of bags of shopping for fifteen minutes?

- Does your heart thump when you climb a flight of stairs?

- Do you suffer from all-over aches and pains when you dig in the garden?

- Are you tired after eight hours of mental work?

- Are you very tired after two hours of housework or gardening?

- Do you tend to avoid physical effort if you can?

- Are you left gasping for breath if you run a short distance?

- Is it difficult to stretch up to reach for something on a high shelf or to bend over to tie a shoe?

- Do you frequently suffer back pain?

If your answer is 'yes' to any of these questions, more exercise will positively benefit you.

It is important to determine your general level of fitness before you begin any exercise programme, not only to ensure that it is safe for you to take up, but also because the programme you choose will depend on how much fitness is already 'in there'.

Try walking up and down a flight of fifteen steps quickly three times. If you are reasonably fit you should be able to do this without becoming breathless. If you do become breathless after only one, don't continue – you must be very careful to start any new programme for exercise at a basic level and progress slowly.

Do you need a medical examination?

The Royal College of Physicians and the British Cardiac Society state that 'most people don't need a medical examination before starting an exercise programme'. There are no risks in regular rhythmic exercise as long as the programme begins gently and only gradually increases in vigour.

However, before embarking on any vigorous exercise programme you should consult your doctor if:

- You suffer from bronchitis, asthma or other chest troubles or chest pain.
- You have ever had heart disease or high blood pressure.
- You are still recuperating from a recent illness.
- You have dizzy spells or often feel faint.
- You have joint problems such as arthritis.
- You have frequent oedema (water retention) at the ankles and/or wrists.
- You are concerned that exercise might affect your wellbeing in any other way.

What to expect at a medical

There are specific tests which attempt to determine your suitability for an exercise programme. They are usually available in sports medicine clinics and include an examination of your cardiovascular system, muscles and joints. Your blood is analysed for *cholesterol* and *triglycerides* and your blood pressure is taken as well.

A resting ECG is usually given and sometimes

the ECG stress test as well. For this you pedal a stationary bicycle (a bicycle ergometer) and walk or run on a treadmill in the laboratory, or climb up and down on a bench while ECG equipment monitors your heart.

The oxygen-count

You may also be asked to breathe into a one-way valve which tells the doctor or physiologist how much oxygen is used during the activity you are performing. This oxygen is measured in litres per minute and then expressed as millilitres of oxygen per kilo of total body weight. The oxygen-count gives the tester a fairly accurate measurement of your *aerobic capacity* – the rate at which you use oxygen. This kind of testing is particularly useful if you are recovering from a heart attack or you are very unfit to begin with.

Heart recovery rate – a measure of fitness

A number of researchers use simpler ways to test cardio-respiratory endurance and to measure fitness levels, based on how quickly your heart recovers after exercise. The critical period of recovery is in the first minute after the end of exercise. Measuring your heart recovery rate immediately on stopping your activity and then exactly one minute afterwards will give you a good indication of your fitness level. Your recovery rate is pretty easy to measure for yourself once you get the hang of it.

Check your heart

After exercising for five or ten minutes take your pulse immediately by placing three fingers of one hand on the underside of the opposite wrist where you can feel a throb of an artery. Count your pulse for 15 seconds and multiply by 4 to give you your minute pulse-rate. Take your pulse again *exactly* one minute later and again record your minute pulse-rate. Now subtract the second number from the first to get your recovery rate and indicate your level of fitness.

Recovery Rate Formula:

Immediate pulse - 1 Minute Pulse = Recovery Rate ÷ 10 = Level of Fitness

If the number you get is high then your heart is recovering well and is strong. For instance, if your immediate pulse was 140 beats per minute and 1 minute later it was 100 then

$$140 - 100 = 40.40 \div 10 = 4.$$

This is an indication of a good level of fitness.

Less than 2	Poor
2–3	Fair
3–4	Good
4–6	Excellent
More than 6	Superb!

What Kind of Exercise?

There are several different kinds of exercise: *aerobic, anaerobic, isometric,* and *isotonic.* Each can be useful but probably the most beneficial for overall health and vitality – if you only do one kind – is aerobic. The name 'aerobic' was popularized by Kenneth and

Mildred Cooper in their books *Aerobic* and *Aerobic for Women*. It means 'living, acting, or occurring in the presence of oxygen'. What makes aerobic activities different from all other kinds of exercise is that they demand your body's efficient use of oxygen throughout the whole time you are doing them.

Aerobic movement

Oxygen is the ignition factor in the burning of energy from the foods you eat. A good supply is always necessary for your body's metabolic processes to take place efficiently. When your cells (particularly the cells of your brain) have an adequate supply, you feel well, have stamina, and don't tire easily. If you tend to feel tired often, get depressed easily, or have trouble thinking clearly, it is likely that your body is not getting all the oxygen you need. In short, you are physically *unfit*.

Unfit people find themselves breathless after climbing stairs, lack concentration when they get involved in a demanding mental task, and are often too weary in the evening to do anything but plonk themselves in front of a television set. They also tend to rely on stimulants or depressants such as alcohol to relax or to keep going.

Taking aerobic exercise changes all that. Any sustained rhythmic movement that puts constant demand on your heart, raising your pulse-rate to between 120 and 160 beats a minute, and continues to develop your lung capacity will bring about a number of important changes in your body.

Aerobic exercise can:

- tone your muscles and improve your circulation.

- increase the number and the size of the blood vessels that carry blood from your heart all over the body so you will have better transport of oxygen.

- strengthen your chest wall, making you breathe more easily, as air will come in and out of your lungs with less effort. Soon your body will become capable of taking in far more oxygen than it could before. This oxygen will generate energy for sustaining mental and physical effort.

- make your bones, joints, and ligaments stronger so they have a natural resistance to injury.

- increase the level of enzymes and energy-rich compounds in your body. You will be better able to assimilate and make use of nutrients from your foods. With regular exercise you will find your whole 'system' works better.

- make your body more efficient. And as the efficiency of your heart increases you pump more blood with each beat and your basic pulse-rate will decline.

Anaerobics

Anaerobic exercise, such as running a hundred-yard dash or gymnastics, involves a high level of effort sustained over only a short period of time. The effort is such that during the activity you run into 'oxygen debt', which means that you use up more oxygen than you take in. This is the opposite of an aerobic activity where, once you are relatively fit, you are able to process oxygen efficiently enough to continue running or bicycling for hours without incurring any oxygen debt. Anaerobic activities can be useful for developing muscle tone and power and for training your body to produce great bursts of strength and movement, but an anaerobic activity cannot be sustained long enough to be of real value to your lungs and heart and so to overall fitness.

Isometrics

Isometric exercises are those you do without any actual movement in your joints. They are muscle-tensing exercises. All isometric exercises are based on the idea that you push or pull against objects that are immovable. Tensing muscles in this way brings about an increase in their size in the same way that weight-lifting does, for whenever a muscle is put under strain it gradually increases in endurance and bulk. Isometric exercises are often 'sold' to people on the grounds that they are effortless – the lazy way to exercise. In fact, they do require some energy to perform but nowhere near enough to be useful in building overall fitness. They have a disadvantage, however, for contracting muscles in this static way can cause blood pressure to rise. In anyone with a tendency to heart disease this can be dangerous.

Isotonics

Isotonic exercises such as calisthenics, yoga, dynamic weight-lifting, ballet bar work, and many sports, are more demanding. They call for real movement in muscles and joints and the rhythmic lengthening and shortening of your muscles. For instance, with weight-lifting, when you bend your elbow to raise the weight to shoulder level, your bicep contracts as the tricep at the back of your upper arm lengthens. Then when you straighten out your arm again, lowering the weight, your tricep is contracted and the bicep is lengthened. This kind of repeated lengthening and shortening of antagonistic muscles helps you develop muscle strength and tone and freedom of movement in your joints. It is also useful in correcting a muscle area, such as the abdomen or the upper leg, that has become flaccid and flabby. Some isotonics, such as yoga or stretching exercises, are also important for developing flexibility and suppleness.

Combined exercise

The best total exercise programme you can devise for yourself involves some form of isotonics, such as weight training or stretching exercises done for at least fifteen minutes three times a week, and thirty minutes of aerobic activity, also done at least three times a week. You can alternate doing aerobics one day and isotonics the next if you like. Unless you are determined to become an athlete and the particular sport you have chosen demands work in isometrics or anaerobics, you need not worry about them.

What Kind of Exercise is Best?

Your aerobic activity will build overall fitness, improve your mental and emotional state, and give you energy. Aerobic exercise is the foundation of dynamic fitness. It involves rhythmic movements of your arms and legs and a shortening and lengthening of these large muscle groups. It also puts your body under measured steady stress which builds its strength, stamina and endurance. Rebounding, running, jogging, aerobic calisthenics or dance, swimming, cycling and rowing are all known as aerobic activities since they require large amounts of oxygen and because they make your heart work hard to pump a great deal of blood. Their main object is to increase the maximum amount of oxygen you can process in a given time. This measurement is technically known as your *aerobic capacity*. It depends on how well your body can take in volumes of air and deliver blood and oxygen to all its parts. Since your aerobic capacity reflects the condition of your heart and lungs it is the best indicator of overall fitness.

Isotonic stretching will give you grace and suppleness and will fill in any muscle-toning gaps your aerobic activity leaves, as well as improving the extensibility of your muscles and tendons.

An aerobic activity is not enough on its own unless you choose swimming, which is remarkable in that it stretches muscles all over as well as strengthening them. You will need to do a few slow stretching exercises to increase the flexibility of your joints and balance the muscle work you are doing. Then you will have an unbeatable combination for long-term good looks, health and vitality. The whole routine should take you 30 to 50 minutes three to six times a week. You have to *make* time for it. But the time you make is never wasted, for it will bring you increased energy, mental clarity and fitness so that you will more than make up for it in what you accomplish during the rest of your day.

The principle of overload

The benefits of exercising come as a result of developing strength by progressively *overloading* your body's muscles. Fitness tests are only useful as a rough gauge to determine your present aerobic capacity and therefore just how much *effort* you will need to make to continue to increase your fitness. It is important to grasp the difference between *work* and *effort*. Two people may run a mile in, say, ten minutes and do equal work. But if one raises his heart-rate by 60 per cent and the other only by 30 per cent then their effort has been different. The heart has had to make a smaller proportional response to the load of exercise because of its efficiency. Effort in this sense means the *effort* your heart is making in response to the *work* your body is doing. In order to build dynamic fitness you have to keep up a certain level of effort for a certain length of time. The amount of work you will have to do to achieve this – the distance you will have to cover and the speed at which you will have to run (or swim, or cycle or row) will constantly alter as you get fitter.

chapter 2

Go For It

Until quite recently in human history you simply *had* to be fit or you would not have survived. The life led demanded physical work, movement and activity. The idea of going out for a run or skipping rope would have seemed absurd to someone who spent 14 hours a day in hard labour tilling a field or hunting or protecting his property from possible threats. Now, however, immersed in our world of cars and automation, most of us have to make a conscious effort to use our bodies vigorously. We also have to decide, given the kind of life we lead, our preferences and our purse, what kind of aerobic activity is best to pursue.

Training heart-rate

Whatever form of aerobic activity you choose, it should raise your heart-rate to 60–75 per cent of maximum. This figure, your 'training heart-rate', is easy to determine. In his excellent book on exercise, *Fit or Fat*, the exercise specialist Covert Bailey describes the way to go about it:

● Find your resting heart-rate

Three or four times a day, while you are sitting quietly, take your pulse-rate on the artery near the base of your thumb at your wrist for 15 seconds. Multiply this figure by 4 to get your resting pulse-rate. Add up the figures for several readings collected during the day and divide by the number of readings you have made to get your average resting heart-rate. Then write it here:

Resting heart-rate _____

● **Calculate your maximum heart-rate**
To do this simply subtract your age from 220. This figure will give you an indication of the fastest your heart can safely beat at your age. (You must *never* exercise at this level!) Write it here:

Maximum heart-rate _____

● **Your training level**
Now you can calculate your training heart-rate – the ideal level at which your heart should beat while you are carrying out your biogenic exercise activity. You should calculate an accurate training heart-rate by subtracting your resting heart-rate from your maximum heart-rate, multiplying by 0.65 (i.e., taking 65 per cent of it) and then adding the result back onto your resting heart-rate again. This will give you your training level – the figure you need to remember and to which you must work. Write it here:

Training level _____

Training Level – Example
If you are 45 years old and have a resting heart-rate of 70, then the calculations for your training level would go like this:

$$220 - 45 = 175 \quad (175 - 70) \times 0.65 = 68.25$$
$$68.25 + 70 = 138.25$$

In this case your training level should be below 138 (say 140 for convenience) beats a minute for you to get maximum benefits from your exercise. So when you actually are doing your exercise stop and check your pulse for 15 seconds and multiply by 4 to see that it is at this level. If it is 10 beats per minute (bpm) slower, then you need to make more effort. If it is 10 bpm faster, slow down – you are working too hard.

Getting Started

Whatever aerobic activity you choose – swimming, rowing, cycling, dancing, running, rebounding or any of the others – the important thing is to find the way of fitting it into your life and get busy doing it. Once you have got your routine worked out it is relatively easy to monitor your progress and know when you have to increase your effort to get the workout you need to reach a higher level of physical fitness. You'll be surprised how quickly this happens. Regardless of the kind of aerobics you are doing, the principles are the same.

> You need to exercise *at least three times a week for at least half an hour at a time* and if possible five or six times a week.

Keep it regular

If you can't exercise regularly, you're better off not exercising at all. Working out at weekends or whenever you feel the urge is potentially dangerous, especially if you are over forty. If you are ill or extremely fatigued it is all right to suspend your exercising temporarily, but regularity (at least two, preferably four or five times a week) is essential for you to hold on to the benefits exercise will bring you. If you don't continue working out this frequently, you will lose what you have gained in terms of dynamic fitness.

Go easy

If you find that you rated poor on the fitness test then you will need to start very slowly. Swimming perhaps, or walking, or gentle rebounding. Then you can gradually increase the intensity of your activity to keep your heart-rate at the level which is optimal for you.

Chest Pains – the Danger Signal

If you ever get a sharp pain in your chest, you must stop and seek medical advice *immediately*.

Warning signs:

- Are you short of breath at even the mildest exertion?

- Do you ever have pain in your legs when you walk which goes away when you rest?

- Do you often have swelling in the ankles?

- Have you ever been told you have heart disease?

- Do you get chest pain when you perform any strenuous activity?

What to expect

Once you start any aerobic exercise programme some interesting changes take place. For instance, some people feel fatigued both mentally and physically for a few days. This is because the 'power curve' of muscular strength doesn't rise in a linear way on starting a programme of vigorous exercise. It takes time for your body to adjust to the unaccustomed workload – usually about a week – so that you are in a 'get worse before you get better' situation. It is good to keep this in mind, since knowing it may happen will help keep you from becoming discouraged if it does, and prevent you from leaving off your programme before it begins to show benefits.

The more you exercise, the better your condition will become and the greater will be the rewards. From the first session you will experience a feeling of satisfaction plus a few aches and pains here and there. Very soon, however, you will get into the flow of things and by the end of your first ten days or two weeks you'll find your energy levels steadily rising and your body feeling great. After three months on your new programme you will probably find you don't want to miss a session because you just won't feel the same if you do.

The warm-up
It is important to begin any aerobic exercise (except swimming) with a five- to ten-minute period of slow, rhythmic stretching exercises. There is less chance of injuring a muscle if it is thoroughly warmed up. Doing some warm-up stretching before setting out is particularly important as you get older. Then not only do one's muscles tend to be stiffer and joints creakier, but studies show that in some people a condition where not enough blood gets to

the heart can occur if they launch into vigorous
exercise without a preliminary warm-up. Stretching
exercises not only have a prophylactic effect on your
heart, they also increase your flexibility and help
strengthen muscles which you are not using in your
aerobic activity. The stretches should be done gently
and slowly so your body gradually becomes warm,
yet you are not exhausted at the end of them.

Limbering up

Part of the warm-up is directed at stretching the
muscles at the back of your legs, and strengthening
those in your abdomen and calves. These are particularly important for joggers and cyclists. So the exercises fulfil a double purpose by getting you warm
and relaxed while stimulating the heart and lungs
and filling in any 'muscle-toning gaps' your aerobic
activity creates. Do them *slowly* to prevent opposing
muscles contracting too much, and do them *gently* so
you never damage tendons.

Back leg stretchers

- Sit on the floor with your legs slightly bent and
  lean forward to grasp both ankles. (See that your
  ankles remain flexed so that your toes are pulled
  up towards your torso).

- Now gently push your ankles with your hands,
  bending at the hips and bringing your torso
  and head forward so you straighten your legs as
  much as possible by sliding your feet along the
  floor.

     Don't strain. You can aim to touch your knees
  with your forehead but it doesn't matter much if

you never make it. It is the slow gentle stretch that counts.

- Now, pulling on your ankles, slowly return to the starting position.

- Repeat 10–30 times, increasing the number as you get fitter. You'll notice your thighs becoming firmer.

Special sit-ups

- Lie on your back, knees bent and feet flat on the floor.

- With your hands clasped behind your head raise your torso 6–8 inches off the floor (no more) slowly and smoothly. Then slowly and smoothly return to your starting position.

    These sit-ups are specially designed to bring into play your abdominal muscles. They don't get a full workout in the conventional sit-ups where you are lying with legs stretched out, which tends to put too much strain on the back.

- Repeat 15 times and work up gradually to about 50 times.

Foot twists

- Sit in a chair and cross your legs so one leg hangs free.

- Twist the foot at the ankle round slowly in a clock-wise direction, pulling hard so that the ankle is flexed at the top of the circle and the toes are pulled up hard. If you do it correctly it is quite a difficult exercise.

- Reverse the movement and do it counter-clockwise. Then change legs and repeat. This exercise strengthens the front of the legs and the ankles.
- Do 5–8 circles in each direction for each foot.

There are some other excellent stretching exercises which are particularly good for hips and legs and will help you develop more flexibility of movement all round.

Side lunges

- Stand with your feet wide apart, hands on hips, left knee bent keeping your right leg straight, press the inside of the right leg towards the ground.
- Return to the starting position.
- Repeat ten times then change sides.

Forward lunges

- Stand with hands on hips and feet slightly apart, one in front of the other.
- Stretch as far as you can, pressing your bottom forward towards the ground and bending the knee in front of you as you lunge forward.
- Repeat ten times returning to the starting position each time.
- Change legs and repeat.

Cooling off

Just as you need to warm up before exercising aero-bically, you need to cool your muscles off gradually too. While you are exercising much of your body's blood rushes into the area of muscle you are using. With each movement the contractions in these muscles send the blood rushing back to the heart and the rest of the body. But if you suddenly stop moving, much of the blood can 'pool' in one part instead of being sent back to the brain and the heart. This can result in dizziness, nausea and even more serious problems. You need to take five minutes at the end of exercise during which you slow down to a walk but keep moving in order to help eliminate the waste products of exercise quickly and lessen or prevent the heavy, slightly sore, feeling that can follow it. Especially at the beginning – before you are really fit.

Thinking positively

Nothing can ruin an exercise programme faster than negative attitudes. Yet many of us are stuck with them because we have grown up to consider exercise something you only do under duress in school. Exercise can be fun. Not at first maybe, for it can be hard work when your muscles are soft, your joints stiff and your heart and lungs not used to so much exertion. At first it is natural to feel a little awkward and heavy. But each time you start to work out, let your mind play over all the benefits which it will bring you. You'll find that any original discomfort passes quickly if you just persevere. Remember that many other 'doubters' have already discovered a new, healthier and more exciting way of living through dynamic fitness. Expect this for yourself too.

Freshening up

Once you have cooled off a bit and stopped sweating you will probably want a shower – more invigorating than a bath – but don't make it too hot and try to finish off with a 30-second cold shower.

If you choose to have a bath, be sure the water is warm, not hot. Never soak in really hot water, otherwise you may start sweating again and will feel lifeless and dried up when you get out. When you have washed, try emptying your bath and then refilling it to about eight inches with cold water. Stand in it and sponge yourself down starting with your lower legs and working up to the waist. Then sit down and splash thoroughly your torso and finally your shoulders, neck and head. Finish off with a rubdown with a towel and dress warmly afterwards. Cold water used in this way has an exciting effect on the body. It benefits both blood and circulation, and it tones and promotes the repair of muscles. It also makes you feel really good.

chapter 3

The Joy of Exercise

There have been several studies of the physiology of exercise, and now it is generally agreed that the best sorts for overall fitness are aerobic activities. For only these activities offer the kind of steady, sustained movement that builds muscle strength, increases the flexibility of joints, and also fortifies the heart and lungs.

Swimming

Swimming is one of the best of all the aerobic activities to start with, particularly if you're very much overweight. The support the water gives your body makes you able to put all your effort into participating in the movement, instead of having to direct some at just keeping yourself erect as you do in running. Swimming is also a wonderful way to build beautiful muscles if you are very thin, or to pare down and firm up muscles if you are flabby. This is because swimming develops long muscles in the legs and back, gradually reshaping and reforming any body that has lost its shape, no matter what its age.

You will need to set yourself a goal – say, at first

fifteen minutes of constant swimming from one end of a pool to the other without stopping – and stick to it. If you are troubled by chlorine wear goggles. They will keep your eyes protected. Begin slowly. Swim a couple of laps and then stop and, using a watch with a second hand take your pulse to monitor your training level.

Begin gently. Swim for fifteen minutes the first three or four times. Then you can gradually add a couple of minutes each week until you work up to thirty minutes, three times a week. At this level, provided you monitor your effort by taking your pulse occasionally, you can be assured of gradually and steadily building fitness. However much you do, watch your breathing while you swim. It is important to breathe regularly, for oxygen is what gives you the power to sustain the physical effort you are making. This is what aerobic fitness is all about.

Cycling

The same basic principles apply to bicycling. It too is an excellent endurance sport that promotes co-ordination and muscle strength, particularly in the lower half of your body. The other good thing about bicycling is that it gives you a feeling of getting good return on energy expended, as a bicycle will carry you a lot farther than a run or swim with the same effort.

Cycle in the early morning or on country lanes, then you will be able to keep up a steady pace without having to stop for signals, cars, or pedestrians, and the air is free from dust and fumes. You can take your pulse in the same way – after, say, five minutes of bicycling – to ensure that you are making the right effort. And you can start off with fifteen minutes' bicycling and then work up to half an hour or more three times a week. Make sure that the seat and the handlebars on your bicycle are the right height for you or you can end up with back strain. And be sure to look after your bicycle well so it offers little resistance, for although working against unnecessary resistance from a machine may be physically beneficial when you are using an indoor bicycle exerciser, it can be an awful bore and very discouraging.

Bicycling is a particularly good sport to take up if you have a family, as children delight in going on bicycle outings. An ideal Sunday afternoon activity is to go on a fifteen or even twenty-mile bike ride together, especially if there is a delicious picnic in the middle.

Rebounding

This consists of movements such as skipping, jumping, running on the spot or arm flinging on a firm mini-trampoline called a 'rebound exercise unit'. Rebounding will do all that other forms of aerobic exercise can – strengthening your heart and lungs and firming your muscles – and more, because of the unique way in which your body is subjected to the changing force of gravity when it bounces up and down. Rebounding crosses the generation gap too.

The bouncer units, which look rather like low coffee-tables, consist of a steel or aluminium frame on six or eight legs over which is sprung a drum of firm but elastic material on which you bounce. You can use a bouncer anywhere. With rebounding you can dress in any way you like, watch television, listen to music or carry on a conversation while you are exercising.

Manipulating the force of gravity

From a physiological point of view, what gives rebounding its potency for building fitness, improving health and retarding ageing is the way it makes use of the force of gravity. It is the only form of overall vertical, rather than horizontal, exercise. The upward and downward movement on a bouncer, coupled with acceleration-deceleration, brings about continual changes in the force of gravity exerted on your body. All its organs, the circulatory and lymphatic systems, and even individual cells are affected, in a way that no other form of exercise can accomplish.

The G-force at the top of the bounce is non-existent, as, for a moment, your body takes on the total weightlessness of an astronaut in space. Then when you come down again onto the elastic mat the pull of gravity is suddenly increased to two or even three times the usual G-force on earth. This puts all parts of your body, from the tiniest cell to the longest bone, under rhythmic pressure.

The kind of cellular stimulation the body receives from this continual gravity/non-gravity exposure appears to have remarkable and unique benefits. Waste materials in cells are gently eased out into the interstitial fluid to be carried through the lymph system and eliminated from the body. Increased oxygen is brought to the cells to stimulate cell metabolism. Cell walls appear to grow stronger and cells to function more efficiently with repeated use of a rebounder. This leads to a gradual detoxification of your whole system. The texture of your skin improves, your energy levels rise and sometimes even within only a few days your body begins to look younger and to feel far better. And because rebounding is amusing, it is a form of exercise which even couch potatoes like.

Rebounding for rehabilitation
Using a bouncer regularly can be an excellent way of exercising if your body has sustained some kind of injury, such as a twisted knee or *achilles tendonitis*, while running or doing some other form of exercise. It gives the exercise enthusiast a chance to maintain fitness and still let the injury heal, and helps to avoid the familiar depression that sets in when you cannot exercise.

Walking
Probably the most neglected of all activities that can build health and fitness, walking can be tremendously enjoyable no matter what your physical condition. In many ways it is the best form of aerobic exercise for most people. The rewards are many, varied, and immediate. There are the delights of feeling fresh, pure air entering your body, the tingle of a cold morning, the wind and rain on your face. You can become absorbed in the sights you see. Such things can engage your mind and dissolve your sense of time and thoughts about stressful aspects of your life.

As with most physical activities, the rewards of walking are directly related to the effort you make doing it and to the spirit in which you do it. A gentle stroll without purpose or a grudging constitutional with the dog will do little for you. But taking a brisk walk with good will and a sense of purpose while breathing deeply will put a glow on your skin and help improve your posture, the condition of your muscles all over, and your circulation. If you choose walking as an aerobic activity, make a date with yourself to spend thirty minutes a day at it.

Walkwear

It doesn't matter what you wear as long as it is comfortable and unrestricting. But you do need a good pair of sturdy shoes. They should be stout so that they give you a feeling of security and reliability over even the roughest and wettest ground; thick rubber soles are particularly good because they both grip and act as shock absorbers.

Natural fibre socks are better than the synthetic because they are more absorbent. You needn't be deterred by wind or weather either; walking in the rain, provided you are well dressed for it, can be a delight. A lightweight wind- and water-proof jacket is a great help.

Start off walking briskly – fast enough so that you will be a little out of breath. Feel the rhythmic movement of your body and the way your legs swing freely from your hips. Get into the swing of it all, then after the first week or two increase the time you spend to forty-five minutes and vary your pace. Try not to walk over flat ground all the time – the hills and valleys, the ups and downs are what bring real physical rewards.

Monitor your progress

Walking regularly can bring fitness slowly but surely without ever taking a pulse or timing anything. A walker can measure her progress by self-observation alone. Ask yourself how you feel and compare your performance walking with that of six weeks or a few months earlier. You will notice that very soon you are walking faster and farther. You will also probably notice that work has become less of a burden for you, perhaps that you sleep better, think more clearly, and feel more emotionally balanced.

Another good thing about walking is that no matter where you are living or visiting, there is always somewhere interesting to go. In town there are always parks and recreation areas, and even industrial areas can be fascinating in the early mornings or late evenings when the air is relatively free of pollution.

Running

My favourite aerobic sport is running. One of the main reasons I was determined to try it was that running was the one sports activity I did at school at which I was no good at all. Running my first mile was the hardest thing I have ever done in my life, but now I have been running for fifteen years, covering as much as eight miles at a time, and I have developed a passion for it.

My enthusiasm for running is not all the result of a personal bias, either. There are several objective reasons why running appears to be the best form of aerobic activity for many people. For instance, it is something everybody knows how to do already, so no special training is needed for it. Secondly, it is something you can do anywhere so long as you have a good pair of shoes and a street or a field or a beach to run on. You can run if you live in the city. You can run when you travel – it is simply a matter of tucking your running clothes and shoes into your suitcase wherever you go. Running is also something you can do at any time – during a lunch hour or in the early morning while your husband is still in bed if you have children who can't be left alone. You can even run in the middle of the night provided you wear white (and preferably reflectors) and run *towards* the oncoming traffic.

Simple fitness check

There is a simple way to check yourself out for fitness before taking up running. Walk a brisk two miles in thirty minutes. How do you feel afterwards? Do you have any nausea or dizziness? No? Then, so long as you have no medical condition that indicates caution, you are certainly fit enough to start at the bottom of a slow, graded programme for joggers.

If, however, you have any difficulties on the walk, then keep up this two-mile walk every day until such time as you can do it easily in the half hour before you start running (you will be surprised at how rapidly your condition improves even from daily walking). Don't get discouraged, just keep things up and you will soon be running.

Getting into gear

It doesn't matter what you wear to run, provided it gives you freedom of movement and doesn't inhibit the elimination of perspiration. Clothes made from natural fibres such as cotton and wool, which 'breathe', are much better than those made of nylon. In summer you probably won't need more than a pair of shorts and a cotton vest or T-shirt. Bare legs give you a sense of freedom when you run and help keep you cool. In winter you will need a fleecy lined cotton sweat suit and light sweater. Add a light waterproof jacket or parka when it rains.

When the weather is particularly cold you may need a wool cap or a scarf tied around your head to protect your ears. For night running, wear white or light colours, preferably with reflectors, so you can easily be spotted by cars.

Running shoes

While the clothes you run in can come from anywhere and look like anything so long as they are comfortable, your running shoes are a different matter. They need to be specially designed to absorb the powerful impact of your feet hitting the road 1,600 times with every mile you cover. As soon as possible you should purchase a pair of proper running shoes. They are not cheap but they are an excellent investment, probably the best you've ever made for fitness provided, of course, you continue to *use* them. They should not be too flexible. They should be without studs and they need to have a high-density sole. Some of the best soles are made in microcellular rubber. Some soles on running shoes extend up the toe and heel in order to take the rocking motion from heel to toe that running brings.

A good pair of running shoes enables you to run on roads without risking shin splints or the injuries to your knees or Achilles tendons that are easy to come by when you wear just an old pair of tennis shoes. The padded instep in your shoes is also useful in absorbing the shock of each step on hard pavement. When choosing a pair of running shoes, take your time and be sure they fit properly. There should be enough room inside for your toes to move about. Your heel should be slightly raised as this will help protect you from injuring your Achilles tendon, which can be very painful if you overstretch it. The shoe should lace up with five or six pairs of holes so that when it is tied it will hug your foot comfortably. Ideally, your training shoes should fit so well – they should be comfortable but firm – that they begin to feel as though they are part of your feet.

Training shoes come in all different materials. Light leather can be very good indeed. Nylon dries faster and is easier to care for. Plastic and artificial leathers are not very good because they make your feet sweat.

The question of socks is a moot point among runners. Some wouldn't dream of wearing them and others wouldn't ever go without them. I find socks are useful because they keep your feet and the inside of your shoes dry and protect your shoes from odour. Socks also help to absorb shock.

The Graded Programme

First week

Take a brisk walk of one mile, breaking into 50- or 100-yard jogs when you feel like it. Walk at a steady pace in between the jogs but never force yourself. Fitness is gained by steady work. You only end up with injuries and anguish when you push too hard. Take a look around you and enjoy your surroundings. Explore the feeling of your body in motion.

At first it is hard. Even during the first minute or so of your jog your heartbeat rate will climb and you'll find yourself breathing deeper and faster because your body needs more oxygen to meet the demands being made on it. Once your muscles start warming up, your skin will flush as your circulation increases and you may find a little stiffness in your chest as your muscles expand to enable you to breathe more deeply and fully. These sensations may seem strange to you if you are used to being inactive, but they are simply an indication that your body is responding the way it should to this new experience and are nothing to worry about.

Second week

Walk/jog a mile, alternating about 100 strides of each at a time. After a couple of minutes of jogging you will probably experience an oxygen debt – your body is demanding more oxygen than it is yet able to process efficiently. You may feel as if you can't go on. If it is too tough, then walk slowly for a while or simply stop and wait until you recover. After you have run for a few minutes, your joints may start to feel a bit stiff or sore and your legs may feel heavy, like lead – two more unusual sensations. They are also perfectly normal since you are probably using some muscle fibres and joints in a way they are not used to being used. It is to be expected that you should creak a bit here and there.

Third week
Walk/jog 1½ miles, increasing your jogging intervals to 150 strides with 100 strides of walking in between.

When you are able to run for from six to ten minutes without having to stop and walk, you will experience your 'second wind'. Your running will suddenly get easier and your breathing freer, and you will find you are covering ground more smoothly. Sometimes this second wind stage takes time to get to if you are a new runner. But eventually it will come each time you run.

Fourth week
Jog for a while at any speed that is comfortable for you. If you find you can't make it all the way without stopping to walk, don't worry. However, by now you should be able safely to tolerate a little discomfort. It soon passes.

Fifth week
Run one mile in less than nine minutes.

Sixth week
Jog/run 1½ miles or more. By now you will be over the hump and beginning to feel all the benefits of your perseverance. You will have started to be aware of your body and to be able to listen to what it is telling you. You will no longer need to monitor your pulse. Now you can even begin to move differently,

varying your pace, for your stamina and willpower have increased. You can start to push yourself a little bit further some days and to let yourself go more slowly than normal if you are feeling a bit low. You can trust your sense of things.

Fifteenth week

Play about with your speed and distance, increasing your distance when you want. Try to alternate a long run – say four or five miles – with a short run of one or two the next day. By the end of six months of running you will be able to run easily and steadily for from half an hour to an hour, covering between three and nine miles.

After you have been running for several weeks and are able to run for half an hour or so without stopping, you may experience what runners call the 'third wind'. What happens is this: you keep running until you find your muscles beginning to feel sluggish, your breathing very hard, and your legs a bit heavy. You think you should stop because these sensations seem quite strong. Then suddenly you find all this changes.

Your body becomes lighter. The running itself becomes almost automatic and you feel as if you could go on and on. You get a kind of euphoria, or 'runner's high'. It is with the arrival of this third wind state that many runners experience the meditative aspects of their sport. Your mind becomes calm and clear, your perceptions heightened, your movements fluid and more effortless than ever before. It is a very exciting experience and one which, although it does not happen to every runner, is quite common.

Listen to yourself

The best way to use a graded programme like this is with flexibility, always adapting it to your own individual needs and level of fitness. If in the early stages you find weeks one, two, and three are very easy for you, then you can try a higher level instead. So long as your pulse-rate when you are running lies within a safe range, what you are doing is right for you.

The more you run, the more in touch with your body you will feel. You will begin to notice that once flabby thighs are remoulding themselves automatically. Your posture will get better, your skin will be clearer, your elimination more efficient.

Improved eating habits

Your eating habits will also probably change for the better – slowly and imperceptibly – so you may not even notice until you look back a couple of months later and find that you have no trouble resisting those not very nutritious goodies that looked so delicious a few weeks back. You will also find it easier to trust your body to *ask* for what it wants. Everything seems to work for you more harmoniously and better than before.

Age – no barrier

How old you are, how overweight you are, how out of condition you may be now matters little when you take up running, so long as you follow the step-by-step programme and have your doctor's OK. Where you are *now* and where you will be *then* (in three, six, or twelve months' time) are completely different. Running makes things happen from the *inside*.

Is running dangerous?

In recent years, with greater numbers of people running, there has been an increasing number of scare stories in the press about how dangerous jogging is. You know the kind of thing, about all the people who supposedly suffer heart attacks from running. The latest scare is that running on roads will damage your back because of the jolt that travels upward from repeated impact of your feet against the hard surface. It is true that running can be dangerous if you are very out of condition and you go about it foolishly – that is, without your doctor's OK, without the right shoes on hard roads, and without starting gradually on a graded programme. Otherwise there is no reason to fear that it will harm you.

Word of Warning
Never jog after a meal or a hot bath, or if you are feeling really cold.

The cool-down

Just as important as beginning slowly is how you end your run. When muscles have been very active they need help to cool off gradually. This you can accomplish by walking for five or ten minutes after each run. This keeps extra blood flowing through the muscles and helps your body to eliminate the waste products of exercise such as lactic acid, which can otherwise make you stiff or sore.

During the cool-down you can shake your legs occasionally, do some stretching exercises if you like, such as bending over from the hips, or simply shuffle along at a slow walk for a while.

Persevere

You will probably find, when you first start running, that you have a few aches and pains in your legs, hip joints, or ankles because your muscles are not yet in condition. This will soon change, and provided you are not in great discomfort you can ignore them. Muscle ache passes far more quickly than you would think. In a few days you should not have to deal with it any more.

Troubleshooting

If you get a stitch in your side or your shoulder while you are running, don't worry about this either. Stitches are common and don't mean anything. You can stop and walk if you like, or just jog through it until it passes by slowing your pace a little and breathing deeply. The fitter you get, the less likely you will be to suffer one.

Avoid chafing

Sometimes you get a little chafing under the arms or between the thighs as a result of skin rubbing against skin while you move. You can remedy this or prevent it altogether by applying a little petroleum jelly to the area where it occurs before you begin. (Put some on your lips too if they chap easily.)

Sharp pains

Most aches and twinges here and there are of little consequence and soon disappear. But if you ever have a *sharp* pain in a muscle, stop. You may have torn some fibres.

The pain means that, although you cannot see it, the muscle is bleeding inside, which will make it harden and swell slightly. Put an ice bag or cold compress on the area and get advice from a medical authority on sports injuries if the pain doesn't disappear in a couple of days.

Creating Energy

The experience of gaining energy from running or any other aerobic activity is a common one. You will have it too. And there are things you can do to enhance it.

The *hara* centre

For instance, each day before you begin your activity, try to be aware of your body as an energy factory by focusing your attention at a point a couple of inches below your navel. This is known as the 'hara' centre. If you are able to think of your *Self* as emanating from it – not just when you are exercising but whenever you need energy – you will find this releases a great deal of vitality.

The Oriental influence

This technique is traditionally used for creating powerful yet controlled movements for the Oriental disciplines such as *Aikido* and *Tai Chi*, and even for Japanese and Chinese *calligraphy*. The *hara*, located in the abdomen, has always been considered a centre of power – like a smouldering furnace in which the fire is forever waiting to burst into flame. As you begin your movements, keep focusing on this area and make every movement as though it comes from there.

Find your own pace
When you are running or swimming, bicycling or
rowing, focus on the *hara* centre, gradually increasing the speed and force of your movements until you
find your own pace. It should be one that makes
enough physical demand on you (you can check that
by your pulse), but not so much that you are left
gasping for breath. Then you are ready to get into the
second energy game, that of being *here and now*.

The here and now
Almost everyone has experienced the ability to sum-
mon up energy, almost magically, to cope with particularly demanding situations – getting a second
wind when you have been up all night nursing a sick
child and thought you couldn't possibly drag even
one more ounce of strength from yourself . . . having
an all-encompassing fatigue somehow disappear
into thin air with the unexpected arrival of a much-
loved friend you haven't seen for years . . . discover-
ing the extra strength that an athlete gets at the end
of a long race when he feels he has given all he had.

Are you totally involved?
What, more than anything else, determines how
much energy you have in any of these situations is
not your physical strength, nor what you ate for
lunch, nor even how much sleep you had the night
before. It is simply whether or not you are *totally
involved* in what you are doing – physically, mentally,
and emotionally. This is the theory of biologists,
sports experts, and psychologists who have looked
seriously at the phenomenon of energy or vitality
and tried to distinguish between the traits of those

people with high energy levels and the rest of us. They find that athletes, executives, artists, or whoever, all high-energy people have one thing in common: *total involvement*.

For most of us this kind of complete involvement doesn't come naturally. It probably did when we were children, but it is an ability we have since lost. While you are exercising is an excellent time to relearn it. Here's how.

How to achieve total involvement
While you are exercising pay attention to your surroundings – the sights, the smells, the feel of the air – and to your own inner sensations. Visualize something in graceful motion such as a horse or an antelope, a dolphin or an eagle soaring in the sky, and focus on yourself as a thing in motion. It will give you feelings of strength and grace that will help you keep going.

The whole experience should be demanding but satisfying, not felt to be an awful chore. When you feel you want to stop, do. But be aware of *why* you have stopped. Are you short of breath? Anxious? Did you lose the image in motion? Your reasons will probably be different each time it happens.

Practise this for three weeks or so, allowing your pace and your images of motion to change according to how you feel each day. Sometimes you will go faster. Sometimes you will hold back. That is all part of the process. Simply be aware of what is happening and let it happen. Gradually you will find your body gaining strength, your breathing becoming easier and your movement more graceful. You will find that you are also developing the art of being *here and now* in other areas of your life too. It gets easier and easier with practice. At the end of three weeks you will be bounding with vitality and radiating a healthy glow. And your energy levels – no matter what kind of energy you need, mental or physical – will have soared. That, after all, is what exercise is all about.

chapter 4

The Fully Alive Body

There is no more health and beauty through natural movement than you will get from vigorous aerobic exercise alone. For no matter how far you run, no matter how fine an athlete or dancer you are, unless your muscles and joints move freely through the *full* range of motions possible for them you quite simply won't feel fully *alive*. You will have neither the full freedom of locomotion nor the complete enjoyment of your sensations. You need to teach your muscles to stretch to their limits and encourage your joints to move fully.

This calls for some slow, sustained *isotonic movement* such as yoga or stretching. Practising for a few minutes three or four times a week will not only increase your vitality and your capacity for experiencing joy and pleasure, it will also eliminate the chronic tension that results in headaches.

Aerobic exercise often doesn't go far enough. It does not offer the body enough weight resistance to maintain muscle mass. Exercise physiologists have come to realize that although aerobic exercise has a place as *part* of an exercise programme it does not maintain bones and muscle the way resistance exercise does. The bottom line is that we need both, although resistance exercise is the more important of the two.

Let's Get Started

What does a confirmed couch potato do once he or she decides to explore how exercise can change his or her life? First you get approval from your doctor to make sure that there is no reason you should not start on a simple graded programme. Then go easy. If you start small and work up you will win. If you start big you can not only wear out your body but also lose your taste for movement. The whole effort will then have become counter-productive since you will end up hating exercise and getting nowhere.

For this type of exercise to work it has to become an ordinary part of your daily life. It needs to be done regularly at least three times a week. Begin with only 15 minutes in the morning when you get up or at any other time of the day that is convenient. The great news is that right from that very first session your body will begin to rejuvenate itself. Exercise routines progress well when you work out at the same time each day. Try to do this if you can. Your body will get used to the routine and love it. When it comes to resistance training you don't need to own a lot of fancy equipment either. Nor do you need to join a gym. A couple of dumb-bells will do. Later on, if you catch the exercise bug, you might like to have a barbell as well.

Free weights

Dumb-bells and barbells are what are known as *free weights* as opposed to the kind of gym equipment you find in a multitude of sizes and shapes and glitzy finishes these days. They are also far simpler since you can tuck them under the bed out of sight when they are not in use and you can make use of them any time you want without having to dress in special clothes and go to the gym.

Choose the kind of dumb-bells – each of which fits into one hand – that have six removable weights on each so that you can add and then take off weights as needed for each exercise. Your body and their weight against gravity offer all the resistance you need to work muscles deeply.

The machines you find in gyms are designed to mimic the effects of free-weight exercises but, with a couple of minor exceptions, no matter how flash they look, they are not as good as simple free weights because the range of movement which you go through in each exercise is restricted by the machine. Free weights should form the basis of any good weight-training routine, whether you are a complete beginner or a professional weight-lifter.

There are three things you want to accomplish in your exercise programme. First, you want to maintain and to improve your heart and lung fitness. For this you will use weights plus some form of aerobic activity for warming up and cooling down. Secondly, you want to maintain and increase your muscle mass. Finally, you want to maintain and improve your flexibility and for this you need some kind of slow stretching afterwards.

Warm up
It is important at the beginning of any exercise session that you spend a few minutes doing an aerobic

activity. (You must never pick up a weight when your muscles are cold.) This can be running on the spot, slow steady jumping jacks, using a rowing machine or bouncing on a rebounder. In the beginning your total exercise session may last only 15 to 20 minutes, in which case you will want to devote five minutes at the beginning to the aerobic warm-up. Later on it can be longer.

You could use a rowing machine for about 10 minutes at a slow steady pace to get your heart and lungs moving and to warm up before beginning the weights. As the length of your exercise session grows week by week, until it is ideally 45 minutes to an hour at a time, so will the time you spend on your aerobic activities at the beginning and end of the session and perhaps in the middle too.

Stretch out

After this initial period, which should last long enough so that you feel fully warmed up, you should then spend five to 10 minutes stretching. Stretching before a workout but after a warm-up is done to allow major muscle groups along with associated tendons and ligaments to be gently stretched, ensuring possible injuries are greatly reduced. Now you are ready for your muscle work.

Weights Workout

To work with weights properly you need to split your sessions into different body parts and work one or two body parts per session, leaving at least 48 hours between that session and the next time you work that body part. The muscle- and bone-strengthening that comes with resistance training does not take place *while* you are using the weights. In fact working out stresses the muscles and bones causing tiny breakdowns in the cells to occur.

It is during the *rest* that comes after a workout that new muscle and bone is built in direct response to the piezoelectric stimulation at a molecular level.

Don't overtrain

If you come to the point of using quite heavy weights and training five times a week then it is important to work out each body part only once a week for it can take about 48 hours for the breakdown process to take place and between 48 and 72 hours to build new strong tissue to replace it. Ignorant of these facts, many body builders and weight trainers overtrain their muscles and end up undermining their immune system. Exercising a particular muscle group every five to eight days is ideal for optimum progress.

Keep in control

Ninety per cent of the men and women who use weights let their bodies swing all over the place and, when they are doing an exercise such as a dumb-bell curl, they let the weight just fall back after each movement instead of being in control.

When you do your movements be sure to keep your body absolutely centred with each movement, only using the particular muscle group that is supposed to be working, and emphasize the *eccentric* contraction or return movement, where you are returning the weight to its original position. Resist the movements all the way back. It is the stress placed on your muscles of lengthening again when they are under resistance load that brings about most of the gains in strength you are after. Be sure while you are working out that you drink lots of water between each set and eat plenty of alkaline-forming foods since any kind of exercise tends to make your system more acid.

The cool- down

It is important to spend a few minutes at the end of a weight session again doing some kind of aerobic activity to cool down. How long depends on the length of your weights session. You can go through the same kind of activity you have used in the beginning of your session or even take a brisk walk, but make sure you stay warm by adding an extra sweater.

The stretch-out

Then do some more stretching for a couple of minutes. You will find that your body stretches more easily now since your muscles are full of blood and energized. Go slow and enjoy the feeling. It can be wonderful.

Beginner's Programme

All of the exercises here are classic weight-training movements. They require nothing more than a couple of dumb-bells (the kind that have six weights on each). Start with the lightest weights. You will be able to tell for yourself if something feels right. Never strain. As your body becomes accustomed to the lighter weight you can add a bit more. The object of the exercise is not to use heavy weights but simply to provide your body with enough weight to create resistance against which your muscles do their work.

Each exercise is done smoothly and with complete control both on the contraction of the muscle group and on the relaxation. While one muscle group is working, the rest of the body remains still and centred. Start off by doing only three training sessions a week with one set per exercise. A *set* is the same exercise repeated a certain number of times with a rest for two to three minutes between.

Work up to longer by adding more exercises for each muscle group you are working with and doing one warm-up set of easy repetitions (10–15) followed by a heavier set using a little more weight (5–10 repetitions). Begin with very light weights – just enough for you to feel that your muscles are being worked as you near the end of your repetitions. Then by the time you are ready to add your second set, put on a little more weight until at the end of your repetitions your muscles feel tired.

Session One: Shoulders and Arms
Dumb-bell press 2 x 10
Side lateral raise 2 x 10
Single arm tricep extension 2 x 10
Tricep kickback 2 x 10
Dumb-bell curl 2 x 10
Concentration curl 2 x 10

Session Two: Chest and Back
Dumb-bell bench press 2 x 10
Dumb-bell flies 2 x 10
Single arm rowing 2 x 10
Dumb-bell shrug 2 x 10
Floor hyperextensions 2 x 10

Session Three: Legs and Abdominal Muscles
Dumb-bell squat 2 x 10
Dumb-bell lunge 2 x 10
Calf raise 2 x 10
Abdominal crunch 2 x 10–15
Reverse crunch 2 x 10–15

The result

Each person is in reality two people: an outer person
and an inner counterpart, that is an individual self
that is utterly unique. Each person has a stable
centre of strength and growth. Each inner person
sees the world in his or her own way, has his or her
own brand of creativity, his or her own needs and
desires, and is a law unto him or herself. The inner
self holds the power to create, change, build, nurture
and transform. The outer person is the vehicle for
what the self creates.

When the self is allowed free expression, then
you become truly beautiful for you are fully alive.
Your body is strong, your skin is clear and healthy,
and your movements, speech and actions radiate a
kind of vitality that is unmistakably charismatic
because it is *real*, an outward expression of who you
truly are. Many of the secrets to calling forth this
kind of aliveness are to be found within the body
itself – secrets which are best learned by working
with muscle.

Once you get the hang of it, exercise is like medi-
tation – one of the most mind-stilling activities in
the world. Meanwhile you will find your muscles
and whole body have come alive. Then your muscles

will begin to glow until after a few months your body begins to feel the way it did when you were a child – radiant with life and spirit.

Leslie's Story

I decided to run because I had read all about the psychological benefits of running and because, after several years of being somewhat a couch potato (apart from mountaineering, swimming, and sailing), I felt I needed to get fit somehow but I did *not* want to be seen. Mustering all the courage I could, I made a dash through the front door very early one morning. I went about fifty yards before I felt that I would die from the exertion and had to stop and walk.

It wasn't my legs, it was my lungs – I just couldn't get enough air. I walked on, panting, for another fifty yards or so and then resumed my jog. I found I could sustain the running for just about the distance between one set of lamp-posts, then I would walk between the next. In this way I finally completed my one mile circuit. I arrived home exhausted, dispirited and depressed.

The next day I found a hundred reasons why I should *not* repeat my performance. But something had got hold of me. And when 5 a.m. came around again there I was, with aching hips and ankles, ready to submit myself to the same torture. I did just as badly.

Painful progress

Three or four days later, to my amazement, I found I could run between *two* sets of lamp-posts before having to walk the next set. Ten days later, somehow, streaming with tears I actually ran a mile. I had the same desire to stop and walk several times but for some reason I didn't. I kept saying to myself, 'Just a little farther and then I'll stop' – but when 'a little farther' came I pushed on again and again.

When I finally arrived home, instead of being pleased with my triumph, I had the feeling that I had not really done it. I did repeat it the next day and the day after. Soon I was running two miles a day and then, one wintry morning about six weeks later found I actually *enjoyed* it. I don't mean just the feeling afterwards when you have pushed yourself hard, your face is flushed, and you feel alive and good. I mean the actual running itself. There was something about it that was wonderful to me. I had caught the running bug, which everyone I have ever read on running warns will happen sooner or later, and I wasn't going to give it up.

I've found out a lot about myself and a lot about living from my hours on the road. I have learned that I am capable of succeeding at things I never thought I could accomplish. I have gained a better sense of my own strengths and my own limitations. I have grown thinner, firmer, fitter, and happier. I've rediscovered the fun of play, the idea of doing something for its own sake. Running has also given me more physical and mental perseverance. Perhaps most important of all, I have learned that you have to go through discipline to get freedom.

Two years ago, curious about the transformative effects of weight training I had been hearing about, I decided to try it for myself. I sought out an expert in the field, a Welsh champion weight-lifter, Rhodri Thomas, who was as serious about training as I was about finding out what kind of transformation was possible in the body.

When we began to work I was scared to death. I figured after the first two hours I would collapse in a heap. We worked together six days a week; each day we would work with weights as well as aerobic exercise such as running, swimming and cycling interspersed with other activities such as squash and tennis – just for relaxation.

I was amazed to find that not only did I not collapse but I became fascinated by the process taking place within my body. I watched as muscles I didn't know existed began very slowly and quietly to surface through my flesh. Frequently I found myself pushed to my absolute limits so that the gym floor would be covered equally with sweat and tears. But Rhodri was skilled at his job. He never once pushed me beyond my limits and neither did he allow me to collapse in a heap.

What fascinates me about the experience is not only is working with exercise in this way transformative in that it changes lean body mass to fat ratio and reshapes your body – it also gives you the most incredible radiance, energy and self-confidence. People tell you how wonderful you look, ask you if you have fallen in love, are fascinated by the simple radiance of energy that is present.

One of the inspiring things about this experience has been that some of the ideas about exercise that most of us, me included, have carried around for many years – that you *should* exercise and feel guilty that you don't – seem absurd. Exercise has become a friend, a helper, physical, moral and spiritual support for whatever else I am doing. Where before I often had to exert my will in doing something I now find that that will is supported by a physical strength that I remember from childhood. I think back to all those fairy tales about transformation, about frogs and princes, and for the first time in my life I feel I am beginning to understand what real transformation is about. It is slow and inexorable and it brings gifts far beyond our wildest dreams.

Further Reading

If you found this book useful you might like to read other titles by Leslie Kenton. All are available from good bookshops or simply telephone Murlyn Services on 01279 427203. Titles include:

The Dynamic Health Series: a short series of collectibles on every subject – quick to read, practical and life-changing.

● **10 Day Clean-up Plan** (Ebury Press, £6.99)
A step-by-step guide to regenerating your energy while transforming the way you look and feel – all in ten days.

● **Raw Energy Recipes** (Ebury Press, £6.99)
Eating lots of fresh, raw foods can help you look and feel younger, and protect against colds, flu, fatigue and stress.

● **Cellulite Revolution** (Ebury Press, £6.99)
This plan revolutionizes, rebalances and re-establishes a healthy body ecology so you can live cellulite-free forever.

● **10 Day De-Stress Plan** (Ebury Press, £6.99)
Learn how to master stress with a minimum of fuss and a maximum of pleasure. Start now to make stress a friend forever.

● **Lean Revolution** (Ebury Press, £6.99)
Calorie controlled diets don't work. This book shows you how to eat more to shed fat the energy way.

● **Raw Energy Food Combining Diet** (Ebury Press, £6.99)
Food combining is a smart way to shed unwanted fat without counting a calorie and it will make you feel more alive.

● **Juice High** (Ebury Press, £6.99)
Discover how raw fruit and vegetable juices can energise your life, rejuvenate your body, expand your mind & free your spirit.

The Classic Series: each book a bible combining up-to-date scientific research with the time-tested principles of natural health and beauty.

● **The New Joy of Beauty** (Vermilion, £9.99)
Real beauty is nothing less than the full expression of the individual nature of a woman. *The* bible to health and beauty.

● **The New Ageless Ageing** (Vermilion, £8.99)
A marriage of high-tech science and natural health, this book offers a complete anti-ageing programme.

● **The New Ultrahealth** (Vermilion, £8.99)
The latest research into high-energy health allows you to explore the heights of well-being, physically and emotionally.

● **The New Biogenic Diet** (Vermilion, £8.99)
Health, nutrition and permanent weight loss based on natural fresh foods which have been carefully combined.

● **The New Raw Energy** (Vermilion, £8.99)
This meticulously researched work shows how fresh, un-cooked foods can work wonders for your body and your life.

Also by Leslie Kenton:

Passage to Power (Vermilion, £9.99)
Few women in our culture are prepared for menopause, nor for the next phase of their life. Exploring the biochem-istry and physiology of menopause, alongside myth and archetype, this book will transform the lives of women over 35.

Nature's Child (Ebury Press, £6.99)
How to raise a happy, healthy, independent child the natural way.

Endless Energy (Vermilion, £9.99)
Using simple yet potent energy-enhancing techniques for your body, mind and spirit, learn how to realise your full potential and reach new heights of good looks, creativity and joy.

Index